Anti-Inflammatory Diet

Bid Adieu to High-Risk Health Infections

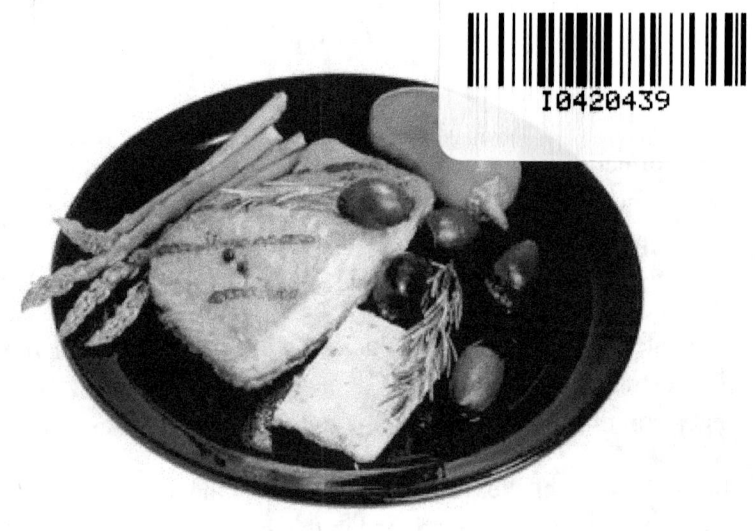

Health Learning Series

M. Usman

Mendon Cottage Books

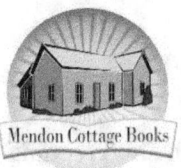

JD-Biz Publishing

Download Free Books!

http://MendonCottageBooks.com

Disclaimer

The information is this book is provided for informational purposes only. It is not intended to be used and medical advice or a substitute for proper medical treatment by a qualified health care provider. The information is believed to be accurate as presented based on research by the author.

The contents have not been evaluated by the U.S. Food and Drug Administration or any other Government or Health Organization and the contents in this book are not to be used to treat cure or prevent disease.

The author or publisher is not responsible for the use or safety of any diet, procedure or treatment mentioned in this book. The author or publisher is not responsible for errors or omissions that may exist.

Warning

The Book is for informational purposes only and before taking on any diet, treatment or medical procedure, it is recommended to consult with your primary health care provider.

Check out some of the other Healthy Gardening Series books at Amazon.com

Gardening Series on Amazon

Check out some of the other Health Learning Series books at Amazon.com

Health Learning Series on Amazon

Table of Contents

Prelude

What does one mean when he/she complains of inflammation? What kind of diet protects the body from harm inflicted by inflammation? Is inflammation permanent?

I'm sure your head is bursting with a multitude of questions regarding inflammation right now; after all it's one of the reasons you are reading this book in the first place! This book will tackle each aspect of inflammation & the diet that is aimed to prevent it, in detail, so relax and ardently enjoy the text that will surely change your life.

Before one can delve into the particulars of the anti-inflammatory diet, he/she has to grasp the biology behind inflammation and it's far reaching effects, as once you get these concepts, you will automatically understand the logic behind the anti-inflammatory diet.

Getting Started

Chapter # 1: Overview

Most people, who are ill-advised on the definition of the word inflammation, consider it a bad thing altogether, while in fact it must be understood that inflammation is a natural response, from the body itself, aimed to remove harmful materials from the body like irritants, bacteria & damaged cells and initiate the healing process. Explained in simpler terminology, when something hazardous tries to or affects a part of the body, there is an internal response from the body to get rid of that entity; this response is inflammation. Inflammation is just a painful swelling, typically red in color, which encompasses parts of the body as a response to some infiltration. The signs & symptoms of inflammation are a measure of the body's progress. Another myth that needs to be busted is that inflammation doesn't mean infection; infection is caused by bacteria, viruses, etc. and inflammation is there to prevent the damage.

Inflammation is part of the immune system and is a healthy response, initially, but sometimes inflammation causes a chain reaction of further inflammations that become self-perpetuating to the extent that they begin to cause more harm than good.

Read on and learn the science behind inflammation.

Chapter # 2: What is it?

Diving a little deeper, it should be known that inflammation is part of our innate immunity. Innate immunity is the body's defenses that are present at the time of birth compared to adaptive immunity which develops after the body is infected and subsequently vaccinated. Inflammation, being an innate immunity, is non-specific and can be a response to a wide variety of incursions in the body.

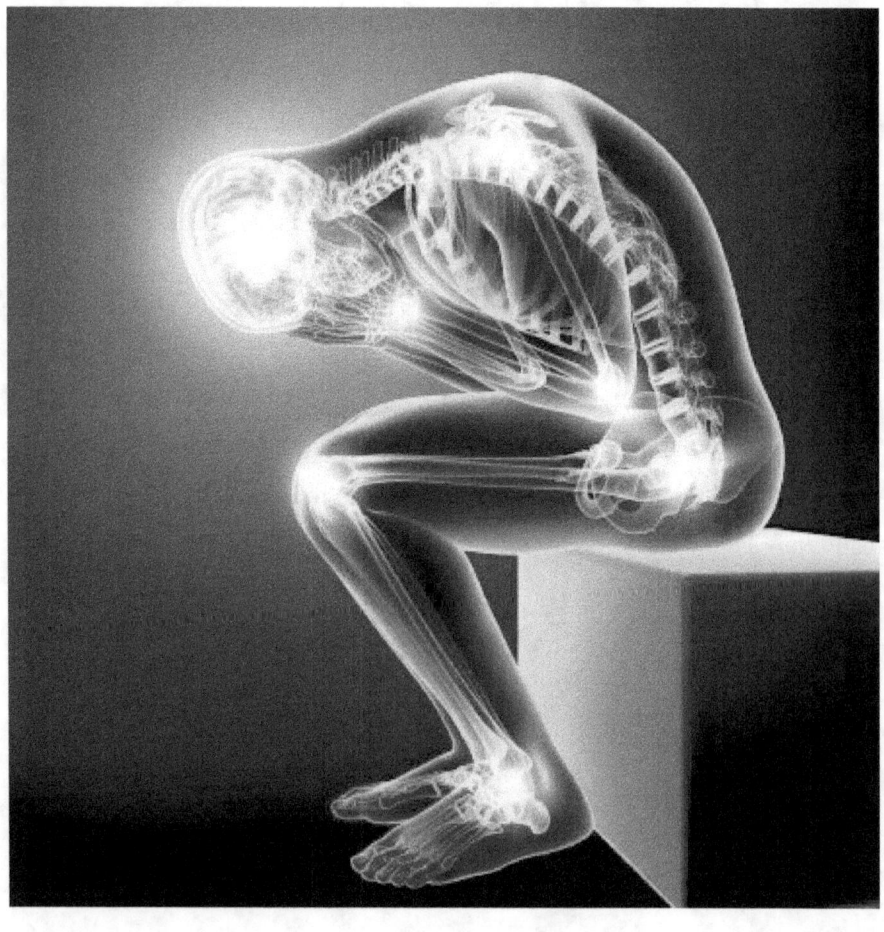

For instance, healing is a process in which inflammation has a significant role. Whenever a person undergoes a swelling, the immediate response of the first aid staff is to bring it down; bearing in mind that inflammation is a required process at this time. The medications written off by doctors are the ones that are absolutely necessary and do not interfere with the healing process.

The healing process aided by inflammation can be divided into three stages.

Stage 1 – Irritation

Stage 2 – The major process of inflammation known as healing

Stage 3 – Discharge of pus

These stages are followed by granulation, which is the formation of masses of tissue on wounds. You see that inflammation is a complex and necessary process without which infections & wounds would never heal.

So what's the problem, if inflammation does well to the body, right? Inflammation can be analogized as a pistol that has a heavy back fire. Initially, inflammation heals the body, but depending on the severity of the disease, sometimes inflammation results in medical conditions that are even worse than the initial one.

There are two types of inflammations that can occur in the body:

1. Acute Inflammation

2. Chronic Inflammation

Each of these types has been explained in detail in the next chapter to prepare you for what's next!

Chapter # 3: Types of Inflammation

Acute Inflammation

This genre of inflammation swiftly develops and rapidly becomes severe, in a race with time! Initially, signs & symptoms remain visible for a few days but lack of care or other conditions can make them persist for a week.

Diseases, situations, and conditions that can result in this type of inflammation include:

1. Acute bronchitis, which is the swelling of the air passages between the lungs and nose.

2. Infected ingrown toenail, self-explanatory!

3. Sore throat or flu.

4. Intense exercise.

5. Acute appendicitis, in which the appendix becomes inflamed or swollen and subsequently gets filled with pus.

6. Acute dermatitis, a general condition that encompasses the swelling of the skin.

7. Acute tonsillitis, contamination of tonsils by bacteria or other infectious agents resulting in swelling,

8. Acute Infective meningitis, the inflammation of the three membranes that envelop.

9. Acute sinusitis, inflammation of the naval cavities.

10. A blow or scratch on the skin.

As it has been previously stated, acute inflammation is swift; within a few seconds or minutes of the injury, physical or one caused by immune response, acute inflammation takes over.

Three main processes that occur at different stages of the onset of inflammation are:

1. Arterioles – Branches of arteries or blood vessels that lead to the capillaries, or smallest branches of the damaged area dilate; this results in increased flow of blood.

2. The capillaries become more permeable resulting in movement of proteins and other fluids in between the cells.

3. Microphages in the blood, like neutrophils, migrate into this inter-cellular space. A neutrophil is a white blood cell that is filled with enzymes that help in digestion and many other processes. Scientists classify these white cells in high regard and consider them the body's first line of defense, but when they show their presence in the wrong place at the wrong time, that's when the problem starts; conditions like heart disease, stroke, and lupus can follow due to the inflammation caused by this cell.

So it can be seen that it is by the third process the body sees real harm; if the body recovers before any stage, earlier than the 3rd one, the body becomes stable; otherwise more complex diseases soon follow

The five signs of acute inflammation include:

Pain – the area that is impacted becomes painful, especially to touch, due to release of chemicals that stimulate pain in a higher amount.

Redness – this is a typical response due to the capillaries becoming filled with blood.

Immobility – in some cases the affected area faces lack of movement.

Swelling – caused by collection of fluid in one area.

Heat – greater flow of blood causes a rise in temperature.

These five symptoms of inflammation are only valid when the affected area is on or close to the skin. When inflammation occurs deep in the body, e.g. an organ, only a few signs are detectable.

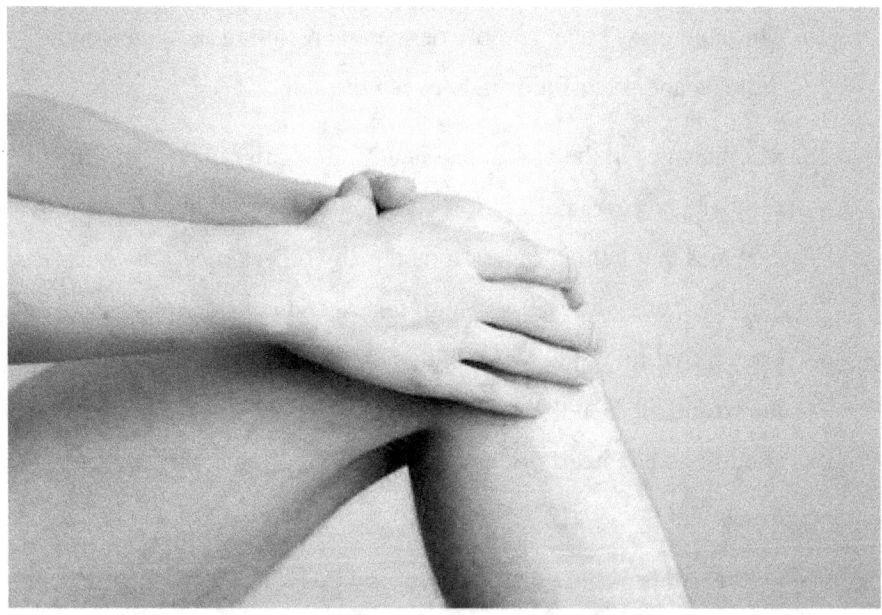

Chronic Inflammation

Chronic means long term or recurring, so by now you should have understood that chronic inflammation is the inflammation that tends to stick to the body for a long time. There are a variety of events, as a result of which, chronic inflammation develops in the body; these include:

1. Failure to eliminate the underlying cause of acute inflammation in the first place.

2. An autoimmune response that results in the destruction of healthy tissues by the immune system, mistaking them for pathogens.

3. An irritant of low intensity that persists.

Diseases and events that include episodes of chronic inflammations are as follows:

1. Asthma, a disease that affects the passage ways of lungs through which air passes.

2. Chronic peptic ulcer, which is a hole in the stomach or esophagus that forms when the lining of the organs are corroded by acidic digestive juices.

3. Tuberculosis, a life-threatening disease that affects the lungs due to infection by the *Mycobacterium tuberculosis* bacterium.

4. Rheumatoid Arthritis, a chronic disorder that affects the joints of the hands and feet, causing a painful swelling that leads to joint deformity and bone erosion.

5. Chronic periodontitis, a disorder encompassing the oral cavity caused by accumulation of dental plaque.

6. Ulcerative colitis, a form of inflammatory bowel disease that is characterized by formation of ulcers in the colon.

7. Crohn's disease, a condition that causes inflammation of the digestive tract or gut.

8. Chronic sinusitis.

9. Chronic active hepatitis, which is a collective term for diseases due to the injury of the liver cells.

So it can be clearly seen that inflammation might be beneficial in the beginning, but wreaks havoc in the body when it becomes long term. In addition to the diseases listed, inflammation can also play a hand in cancers, atherosclerosis and heart diseases, that are all fatal diseases.

A Comparison

Now that both types of inflammations have been covered it's time to examine the difference between the two. The list below describes the major differences between the two, featuring their duration, onset and outcomes.

Acute Inflammation:

Causative agents – Injury to tissue or harmful bacteria.

Major cells involved – Basophils, neutrophils, eosinophils (response to parasites) and mononuclear cells.

Primary mediators – eicosanoids amines.

Onset – Right away.

Duration – Not long, mostly a few days.

Outcomes – The inflammation gets resolved, develops in to abscess or turns into chronic inflammation.

Chronic Inflammation:

Causative agents – Non-degradable organisms that cause a long term inflammation, infection with different varieties of foreign bodies.

Major cells involved – Lymphocytes, macrophages and plasma cells.

Primary mediators – Hydrolytic enzymes, reactive oxygen species, growth factors.

Duration – From months to years.

Outcomes – The destruction of the tissue, scarring and thickening of the connective tissue and death of a multitude of cells.

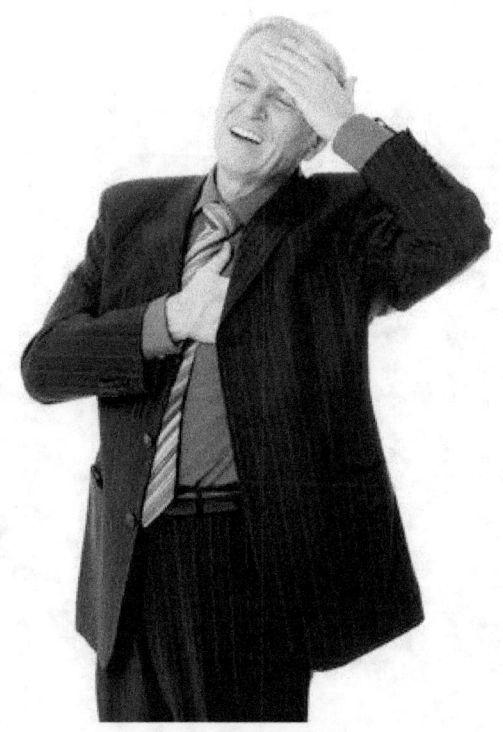

Chapter # 4: Inflammation & Pain

Pain is an entity which has no scale; every individual has his/her own threshold for pain and describes each level in his/her own sensations. People with inflammation often complain of pain, discomfort, stiffness, distress and agony, depending on the extremeness of their condition. The pain felt may be constant, steady or come in intervals, but the general term used for this pain is ache.

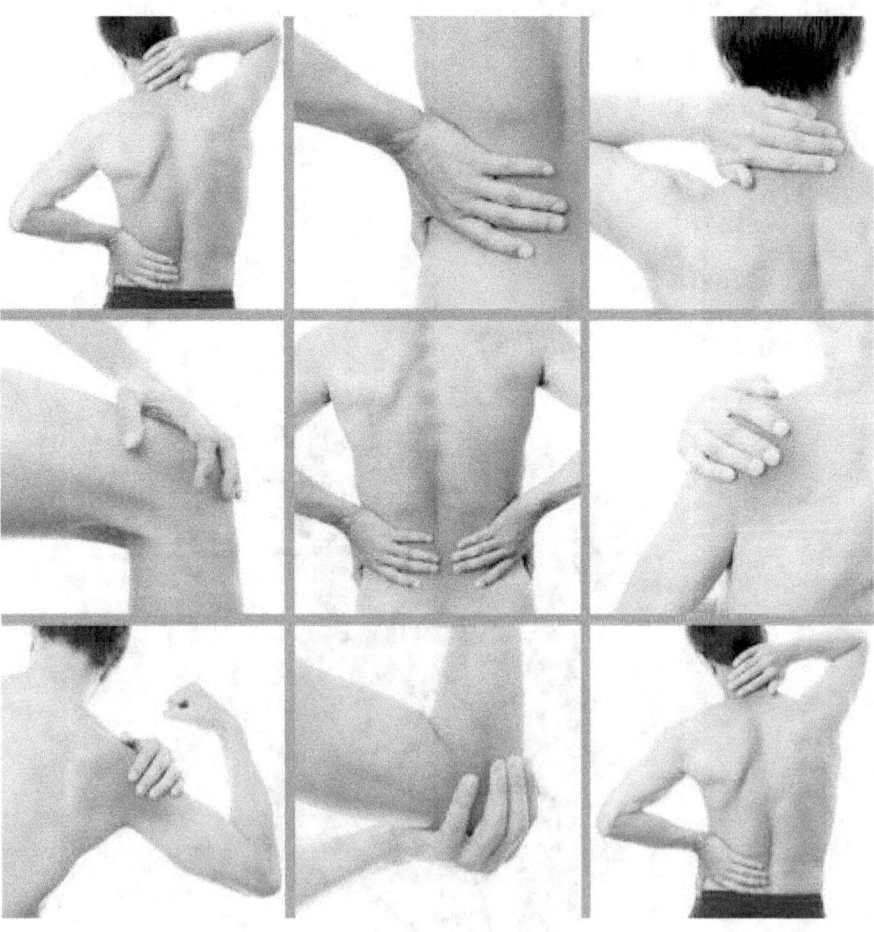

There are three types of pain the body feels while under the effects of inflammation:

1. **Nociceptive pain:**

   This is a general type of pain. In order to feel this pain, specific receptors are stimulated in our body; the response of these receptors change with temperature, stretch, vibration and chemicals released by damaged cells. Nociceptive means reacting to pain – the cause of the pain is not originated from the nervous system and comes from an external source.

2. **Somatic pain:**

   This is one of the types of nociceptive pain; the sensation due to this pain is felt in the joints, bones, muscles, ligaments and skin. During this particular type, pain receptors are sensitive to: stretch in the muscles, temperature, vibration as well as the intensity of inflammation. Somatic pain is usually sharp and much more localized; a touch in the affected area will result in severe pain.

3. **Visceral pain:**

   This pain is sensed deep within the body, like in the main body cavities or internal organs, e.g. lungs, bowels, heart, liver, spleen, bladder, uterus and kidneys. The pain receptors are sensitive to oxygen depletion and inflammation. The pain is not localized and is described as an overall ache throughout the body. Cramping is an example of this type of pain.

Pain is the first indicator for inflammation; it notifies, in an ironically painful way that the body's self-defense mechanism has been activated. Biochemical reactions in the body stimulate pain of different types in the body which tells us about the severity of inflammation and helps decide the further course of action.

When you experience an injury, a number of inflammatory chemicals are released; we won't go into the details of the chemicals involved, but it should be known that these chemicals act as mediators to interact with pain at nerve endings. Long standing inflammations, like arthritis, tend to get a greater response from these chemicals resulting in greater amount of pain in the joints. These chemicals are released at the site of the blow and indicate the inflammation process.

Therefore, keeping all of this in mind, it can be said that in order to control pain, inflammation must be controlled.

Chapter # 5: Inflammation & Living Conditions

Of all the conditions and ailments that affect inflammation, obesity would have been the least expected one on most people's minds, but unfortunately this particularly annoying, yet sometimes life threatening condition, has a profound effect on the markers of inflammation. Men who are overweight or obese have more inflammatory markers in their body as compared to men of the same age who are not overweight; inflammatory markers like white blood cell levels are linked to higher risk of diseases like coronary heart disease.

In a recent study conducted by a team from Pennington Biomedical Research Center in Louisiana, the characteristics of special types of white blood cells were tested with respect to their effect on inflammation. The researchers examined comprehensive test results of each of the subjects linked to their level of fitness, BMI, and adjusted age. The fitness level was measured using METS while the fatness using BMI. (MET is the ratio between the resting rate of energy and working rate) The results showed that:

1. The level of fitness of a person was inversely linked to the level of white blood cells in the body.

2. Men with greater BMI had a raised level of white blood cells in their body.

3. The combine effect of fitness and fatness had a considerable influence on the level of inflammation of the person.

It can be seen that both the factors that affect the level of inflammation can be controlled with a certain amount of effort, therefore, all hope is not lost and there are several ways to maximize control of inflammation.

If the first proof wasn't enough, it has been shown by scientists at the Fred Hutchinson Cancer Research Center, that postmenopausal obese women who lost more than 5% of their body weight had a marked decrease in their levels of inflammation. The results subjected 439 women to a plethora of tests after which it was revealed that inflammation was reduced in women who lost weight with the help of proper nutrition *aided by exercise*.

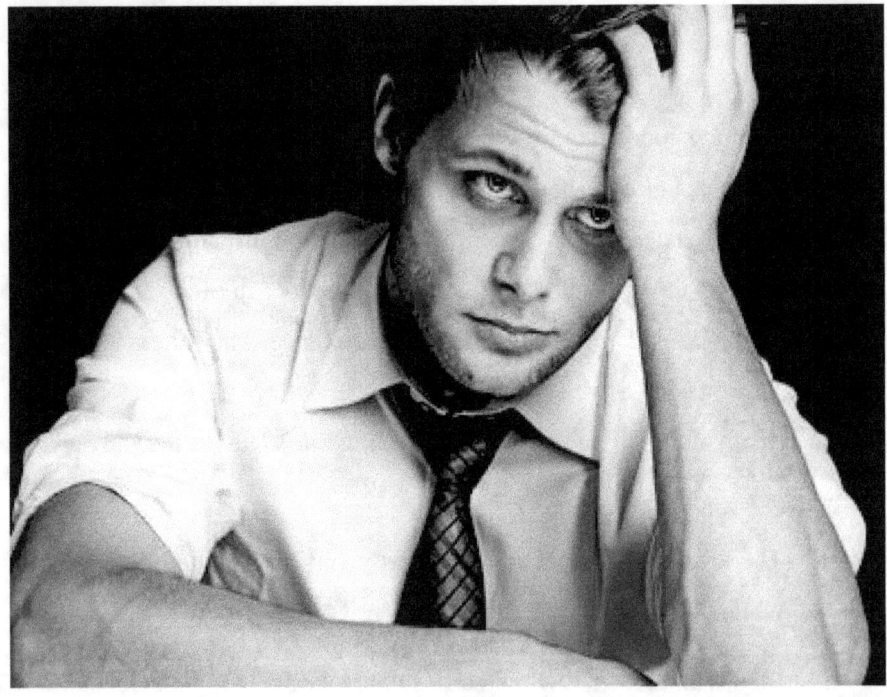

Another living condition pretty much in control of humans that affects inflammation is sleep. Lack of sleep can lead to spikes in inflammation that can, in turn, result in increased risk of heart attacks and stroke. Scientists at Emory University School of Medicine in Atlanta researched and found out that inflammatory markers in sleep deprived volunteers were much higher when compared to individuals who were subjected to normal sleep.

It can be seen that you can positively affect the level of inflammation in your body with your own will, as living conditions are subject to the choices you make for yourself. Get ready to delve yourself in the diet that will get you rid of all the striking pain that halts every daily process in your life.

Chapter # 6: General Guidelines against Inflammation

Inflammation is part of one's life that he/she cannot avoid; what needs to be controlled is the onset of chronic inflammation and its prolonging effect. Controlling what you eat is one the biggest ways by which you can control the level of inflammation in your body, and to some extent, diminish it. Foods that are so quietly and ignorantly consumed by much of the populace are actually a fuel for inflammation markers and therefore harmful to the body. Foods like egg, coffee and bacon might sound harmless, but if looked in a little detail, they cause conditions like cancer, arthritis and diabetes which are all lethal diseases.

The following is a comprehensive, descriptive list of food types one should avoid in order to start alleviating the symptoms of inflammation:

1. **Processed Foods:**

   Packaged, prepared or processed foods often contain ingredients like oils, sugar, sweeteners and additives that fuel the inflammatory process. In addition fast foods can be equally harmful for the body therefore should be avoided to every extent possible.

2. **Hydrogenated & Trans fats:**

   These two substances are abundantly found in margarine and baked products like pies, cookies and buns. Trans fats, which may also be known as bad fats, increase inflammation that wreaks full scale havoc in the body.

3. **Meat:**

Meat, especially red meat, is packed with a high amount of saturated fats which causes inflammation in the body. Meat should be consumed as little as possible by sufferers of chronic inflammation.

4. Fried food:

Once again, fried foods contain a high percentage of fat that is non-beneficial for the body and aids in inflammatory conditions.

5. Wheat products:

It is no secret that wheat available in the market is a genetically modified version and no longer contains the goodness of the original one. One side effect of mutated wheat is that it has high acid-forming ability leading to production of inflammation markers in the body.

6. Dairy products:

Dairy products cannot be defined as a threat to every individual; people who are allergic to these products are the most vulnerable. On consumption of milk, cheese, etc. an allergic person triggers his/her immune system to backfire upon itself and produce inflammation in the body. Hence, lactose intolerant individuals or those allergic to cow milk should at every cost avoid dairy.

At the same time there are several types of food items that do good for the body, calm down the markers of inflammation, and not only are these foods beneficial for the body, they taste good as well. Recipes and specific instructions are given in the subsequent chapters. For now, just have a look at all the good types of foods that have been given:

1. Fatty fish:

Fish are rich in good fats along with omega-3 fatty acids, which are very beneficial for the overall health of the body and not just with respect to inflammation. Examples include salmon, tuna and mackerel.

2. Whole grains:

Whole grains are fiber rich, low additive foods that reduce levels of harmful proteins in the body thereby reducing inflammation.

3. Nuts:

Nuts like almonds, walnuts and peanuts are rich sources of calcium, vitamin E, fiber and anti-oxidants which repair the loss done by inflammatory conditions. Therefore, inclusion of these products in your diet is highly recommended.

4. Leafy vegetables:

Rich sources of anti-oxidants also include leafy vegetables like spinach, broccoli and kale. These vegetables reduce the levels of molecules that support inflammation and, hence, aid in the healing process.

5. Tomatoes:

A chemical in tomatoes known as "lycopene" has the ability to lower inflammation in all parts of the body, especially the lungs. Thus, it is highly recommended that you incorporate tomatoes in your life as much as possible.

Chapter # 7: Five Day Diet Plan

Day 1

Breakfast – Cherry Quinoa Porridge

Makes: 2 servings

Prep time: 5 minutes

Cooking time: 15 minutes

Tip: Add tart cherries if you are suffering from arthritis.

Ingredients:

- 1 cup water

- ½ cup dry quinoa

- ½ teaspoon vanilla extract

- ½ cup dried unsweetened cherries

- ¼ teaspoon ground cinnamon

Directions:

In a saucepan of medium size, stir together all the ingredients, heating to medium heat as you do so. Reduce the heat and let the water simmer for 15 minutes until all the quinoa turns tender. Finally, serve drizzled with honey if desired.

Lunch – Pumpkin Soup

Makes: 8 servings

Prep time: 20 minutes

Cooking time: 35 minutes

Tip: Add pumpkin to reduce symptoms of arthritis.

Ingredients:

- 1 cup chopped onion

- 1 clove garlic

- 1 1-inch piece gingerroot

- 4 cups pumpkin puree

- 6 cups vegetable stock

- 1 teaspoon salt

- ½ teaspoon chopped thyme

- 1 teaspoon chopped parsley

- 1 teaspoon salt

Directions:

Put a pot over medium heat and toss in the garlic, onions and ginger along with ½ cup of stock and cook for 5 minutes. Add pumpkin, thyme, the remaining stock, and salt and cook for 30 minutes. Puree the soup until it smoothens and stir it. Serve along with chopped parsley.

Dinner – Poached Eggs with Curried Vegetables

Makes: 4 servings

Prep time: 10 minutes

Cooking time: 30 minutes

Ingredients:

- 2 teaspoon virgin olive oil

- 2 cloves garlic

- 1 large onion

- 1 tablespoon curry powder

- 2 medium sized zucchinis

- ½ pound button mushrooms

- 1 medium-can chickpeas, drained

- 1 cup water

- ½ teaspoon white vinegar

- 4 large eggs

Directions:

Place a large skillet over medium heat. Sauté the onions until they turn tender and then add garlic, cooking the mixture for 30 seconds. Stir in curry powder until it turns fragrant. Add mushrooms and cook them until they turn tender; add chickpeas, zucchini, red pepper and water and bring the mixture to boil. Reduce the heat, letting it simmer for 20 minutes. In the meantime, pour water 3 inches deep in a sauce pan and boil it. Add vinegar and reduce the heat. Crack eggs and slip them into water, one by one and let the water simmer for 5 minutes. Remove the eggs with a spoon and serve.

Day 2

Breakfast – Raspberry Green Tea Smoothie

Makes: 2 servings

Prep time: 5 minutes

Cooking time: 0 minutes

Ingredients:

- 1 ½ cups chilled green tea

- 2 cups unsweetened, frozen raspberries

- 1 tablespoon honey

- 1 banana

- ¼ cup protein powder

Directions:

Place all the ingredients in a blender and puree until the desired level of smoothness!

Lunch – Kippers Salad

Makes: 4 servings

Prep time: 15 minutes

Cooking time: 0 minutes

Ingredients:

- ½ cup reduced mayonnaise

- 1 celery stalk

- 1 small onion

- 1 tablespoon fresh parsley

- 1 clove garlic

- 1 teaspoon lemon juice

- 1/8 teaspoon salt

- 1/8 teaspoon black pepper

- 1 can kippers

Directions:

In a medium sized bowl, stir together the first 8 ingredients and combine flaked kippers with them. Refrigerate as long as desired.

Dinner – Turkey Chili

Makes: 6 servings

Prep time: 20 minutes

Cooking time: 60 minutes

Ingredients:

- Vegetable cooking spray

- 1 tablespoon garlic

- 1 large onion

- 1 ½ pounds ground turkey

- 1 can canned tomatoes

- 2 cups water

- 1 can canned kidney beans

- 2 teaspoons turmeric

- 2 tablespoons chili powder

- 1 teaspoon dried oregano

- 1 teaspoon hot sauce

- 1 teaspoon ground cumin

Directions:

In a large pot sprayed with oil, cook onions until they turn brown and add garlic and turkey, stirring them frequently until they are fully cooked. Add water and remaining ingredients and reduce the heat; let the water simmer for 30 minutes, and you're done.

Day 3

Breakfast – Gingerbread Oatmeal

Makes: 1 serving

Prep time: 5 minutes

Cooking time: 5 minutes

Ingredients:

- 1 cup water
- ¼ cup unsweetened cherries
- ½ cup oats
- 1 teaspoon ground ginger
- ¼ teaspoon ground nutmeg
- ½ teaspoon ground cinnamon
- 1 tablespoon molasses
- 1 tablespoon flaxseeds

Directions:

Combine the first six ingredients in a saucepan over medium heat and bring the mixture to a boil; let it simmer for 5 minutes and add flaxseeds. After 5 more minutes serve with drizzled molasses.

Lunch – Roasted Chicken Wraps

Makes: 6 servings

Prep time: 25 minutes

Cooking time: 0 minutes

Ingredients:

- ½ cup mayonnaise

- 2 tablespoon pickle juice

- 1 ½ cups shredded cabbage

- 1 teaspoon black pepper

- 1 tablespoon apple cider vinegar

- ¼ teaspoon kosher salt

- ¼ teaspoon pepper

- 1 deli-roasted chicken

- 6 whole wheat flatbreads

Directions:

Combine the pickle juice, mayonnaise and pepper in a large bowl and in a medium bowl add vinegar, salt and cabbage, tossing the bowl as you add each ingredient. Remove and discard bones & skin from the chicken and shred it to tiny pieces; add it to the mayonnaise mixture and stir thoroughly. Divide cabbage mixtures and chicken evenly into the bread slices and roll them; serve.

Dinner – Brazil Nut-Crusted Tilapia

Makes: 6 servings

Prep time: 10 minutes

Cooking time: 10 minutes

Ingredients:

- ¼ cup roasted brazil nuts

- 2 tablespoons Parmesan cheese

- ½ cup bread crumbs

- 1 ½ pounds tilapia fillets

- ¼ cup mustard

- Vegetable spray

- 1 clove garlic

- 1 tablespoon sesame oil

- 1 ½ heads kale

- 2 tablespoons sesame seeds

- ¼ teaspoon kosher salt

Directions:

Preheat an oven to 400 degrees Fahrenheit and lightly grease a baking sheet. Place the Brazil nuts in a food processer and grind them; transfer them to a small bowl and stir in the breadcrumbs. Place the fillets on a baking sheet and spread evenly; divide the nuts in the mixture and lightly spray the crumbs with cooking spray. Bake for 10 minutes. Meanwhile, heat a steel skillet and add sesame oil, garlic (after 15 seconds) and chopped kale. Cook while stirring frequently until the kale turns tender and add sesame seeds; serve the fish with kale.

Day 4

Breakfast – Ginger Apple Muffins

Makes: 12 serving

Prep time: 10 minutes

Cooking time: 20 minutes

Ingredients:

- 2 cups all-purpose flour

- 1 tablespoon baking powder

- 2/3 cups sugar

- ½ teaspoon salt

- 1 teaspoon ground cinnamon

- ¾ cup unsweetened almond milk

- ½ cup mashed banana

- 1 cup shredded apple

- 1 tablespoon apple cider

- ½ cup ginger

Directions:

Preheat an oven to 400 degrees Fahrenheit and lightly grease a 12 cup muffin pan. Whisk together the first six ingredients in a medium bowl. In another bowl, add the next four ingredients and the flour mixture and fill the muffin cups. Finally bake them for 20 minutes and serve after cooling.

Lunch – Persimmon and Pear Salad

Makes: 2 servings

Prep time: 10 minutes

Cooking time: 0 minutes

Ingredients:

- 1 teaspoon whole grain mustard
- 3 tablespoons virgin olive oil
- 2 tablespoons fresh lemon juice
- 1 minced shallot
- 1 teaspoon garlic
- 1 ripe persimmon
- 1 ripe red pear
- ½ cup chopped pecans
- 6 cups spinach, baby

Directions:

In a large bowl, whisk together the first five ingredients followed by persimmon and the remaining ingredients.

Dinner – Red Pepper & Turkey Pasta

Makes: 8 servings

Prep time: 10 minutes

Cooking time: 20 minutes

Ingredients:

- 3 tablespoons virgin olive oil
- 3 large red bell peppers
- 2 teaspoons minced garlic
- 1 chopped large onion
- 2 tablespoons fresh oregano
- 1 tablespoon red wine vinegar
- 2 pounds cooked rigatoni
- 2 pounds ground turkey

Directions:

Cut peppers in half and remove their seeds & stem. In a large oven, heat the oil and add peppers and onion, let them cook for 2 minutes and add garlic. Cooking the mixture for another 5 minutes, transfer the mixture to a food processor and puree it. Return the sauce to a pan and reheat over medium heat. Toss in the oregano and vinegar. In the meantime, sauté turkey in a skillet until it turns brown; let the turkey simmer for 20 minutes and serve over hot pasta.

Day 5

Breakfast – Buckwheat and Quinoa Granola

Makes: 6 serving

Prep time: 20 minutes

Cooking time: 45 minutes

Ingredients:

- 3 tablespoons honey
- 3 tablespoons coconut oil
- ¼ teaspoon ground cinnamon
- 1 teaspoon vanilla extract
- ¼ teaspoon ground ginger
- 1 cup buckwheat
- 1 cup cooked quinoa
- ½ cups old fashioned oats
- ½ cup dried cranberries

Directions:

Preheat an oven to 325 degrees Fahrenheit and lightly grease a baking sheet with parchment paper. In a small bowl, stir the first five ingredients along with oats, quinoa and buckwheat; add honey and spread in even layers on the baking sheet. Bake for 40 minutes; remove and stir in the cranberries and cool the dish before serving it.

Lunch – Roasted Sweet Potato Soup

Makes: 2 servings

Prep time: 10 minutes

Cooking time: 0 minutes

Ingredients:

- 2 ½ pounds sweet potatoes
- ¼ teaspoon kosher salt
- 1 tablespoon virgin olive oil
- ½ teaspoon cracked pepper
- 1 ½ cups sliced onions or leeks
- 1 1-inch ginger
- ½ cup dry white wine
- 1 teaspoon minced garlic
- 5 cups vegetable broth
- 1 teaspoon fresh thyme leaves
- 2 cups orange juice

Directions:

Preheat an oven to 400 degrees Fahrenheit. Cut the sweet potatoes into 1 inch pieces and toss some olive oil, salt & pepper on a baking sheet. Place in an oven for 50 minutes until the potatoes become well browned. In a Dutch oven, cook leeks over medium heat until tender. Stir in the garlic & ginger and cook for a minute. Add wine and bring to a boil. Cook until the wine evaporates and stir in the sweet potatoes, thyme and bring the new mixture to boil; reduce heat and simmer for 30 minutes.

Dinner – Steamed Salmon

Makes: 4 servings

Prep time: 10 minutes

Cooking time: 10 minutes

Ingredients:

- 1 thinly sliced onion
- 1 thinly sliced lemon
- 2 thinly sliced zucchinis
- 1 cup white wine
- 4 salmon fillets
- ½ cup water
- ¼ teaspoon kosher salt
- ¼ teaspoon pepper

Directions:

Place onion and the next 4 ingredients in a large Dutch oven; season the fish with salt & pepper and fit a lightly greased rack over the vegetables you just placed in the oven. Place the water over medium heat until the liquid boils. Reduce the heat to low and place the fish on the rack, steaming it for 10 minutes. Serve the fish on top of vegetables along with sliced olives.

Conclusion

What may start as an indicator to pain and initiator to the healing process, can soon turn into a medical condition that can very likely turn lethal! Once you know how to make a machine, you can easily break it; this is what has been done in this book and that is exactly how you should follow it. First the definition & description of inflammation is given followed by ways to prevent it, thus ensuring that no stone goes unturned. There are surely other ways by which inflammation can be curbed, like taking in medications but so far natural ways have overtaken artificial ones due to their zero side-effects characteristics. A comprehensive meal plan has been included in the book along with "what not to eat" so you would have maximum chance of reversing the effects of inflammation.

Just follow the book and you won't regret it!

Good Luck…

References

http://www.123rf.com/photo_21982629_grilled-salmon-steak-on-plate-served-with-olives-asparagus-and-bell-pepper-isolated-on-white-backgro.html?term=AntiInflammatory%20Diet

http://www.123rf.com/photo_15482591_male-all-joints-pain-in-blue.html?term=inflammation

http://www.123rf.com/photo_27283492_knee-pain-in-men-on-gray-background.html?term=acute%20inflammation

http://www.123rf.com/photo_28243027_pain-in-a-man-s-body-isolated-on-white-background-collage-of-several-photos.html?term=pain

http://www.123rf.com/photo_28068803_stock-vector-allergy-reactions-of-animal-food-environment-on-human-stick-figure-pictogram-icon-cliparts.html?term=food%20inflammation

http://www.fotolia.com/id/48701190

http://www.fotolia.com/id/50889876

Author Bio

Muhammad Usman is a distinguished medical graduate of Allama iqbal medical college (AIMC). He is a professional writer who has been in the field for more than 4 years. During this time he has produced 10,000+ articles, blogs and eBooks on various niches related to diseases, health, fitness, nutrition and well-being. He is a regular contributor to several journals related to medicine and surgery. He is the editor of several journals and newspapers.

Check out some of the other JD-Biz Publishing books

Gardening Series on Amazon

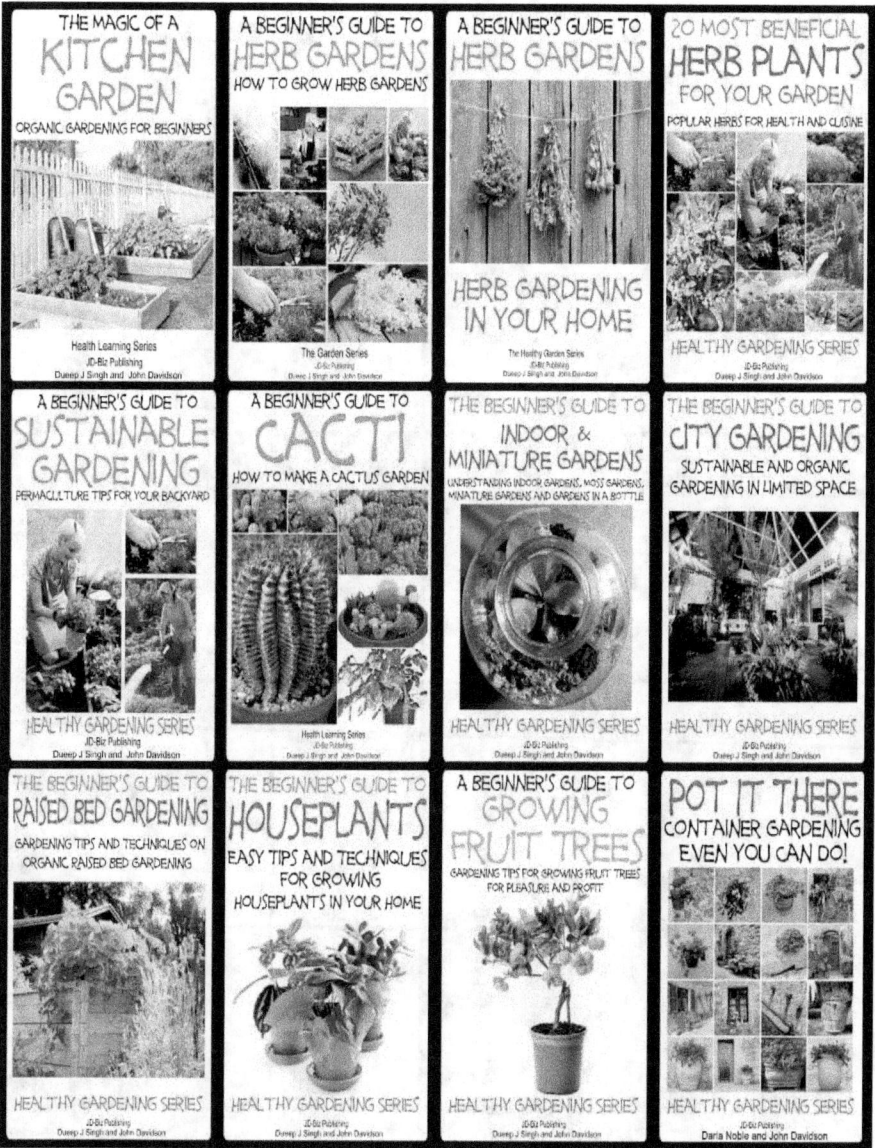

Health Learning Series

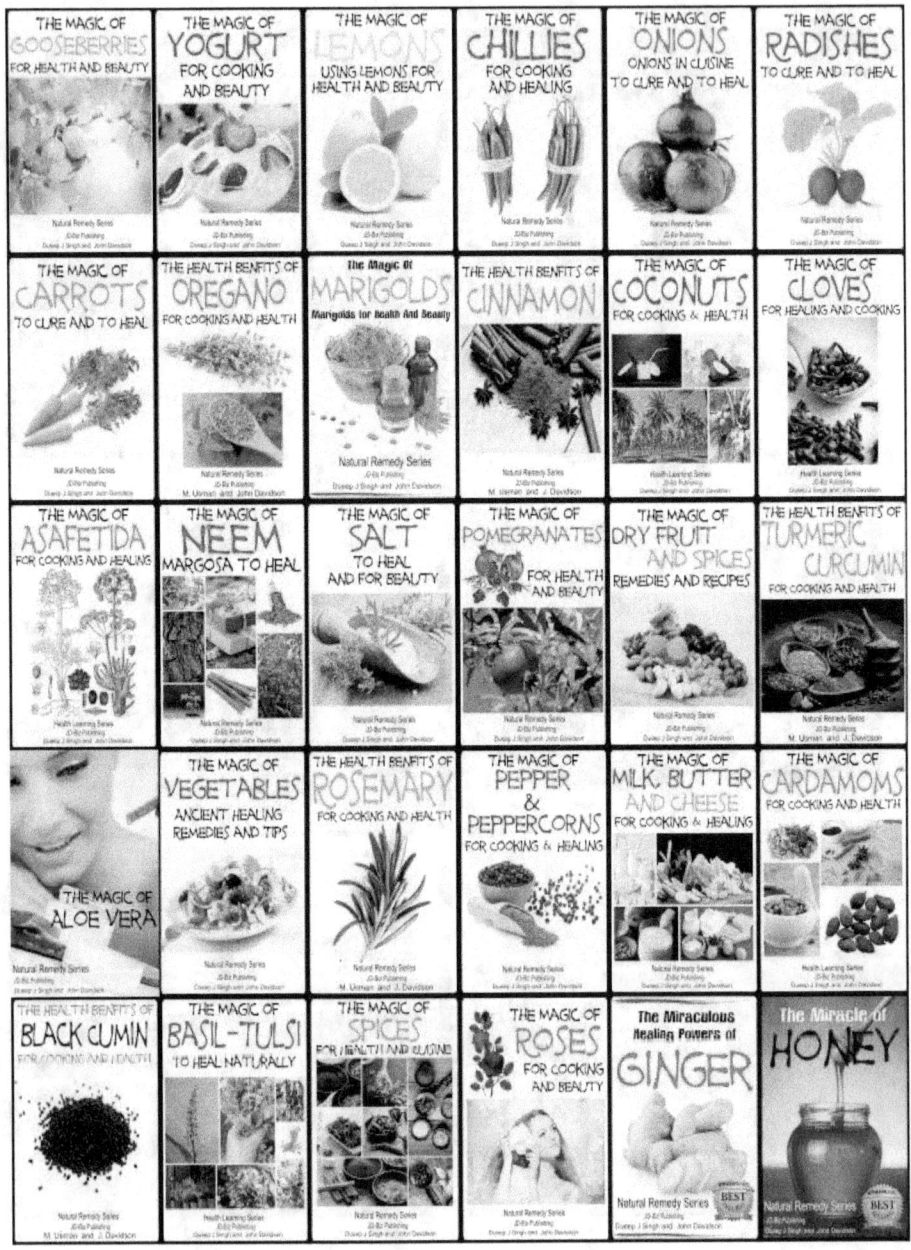

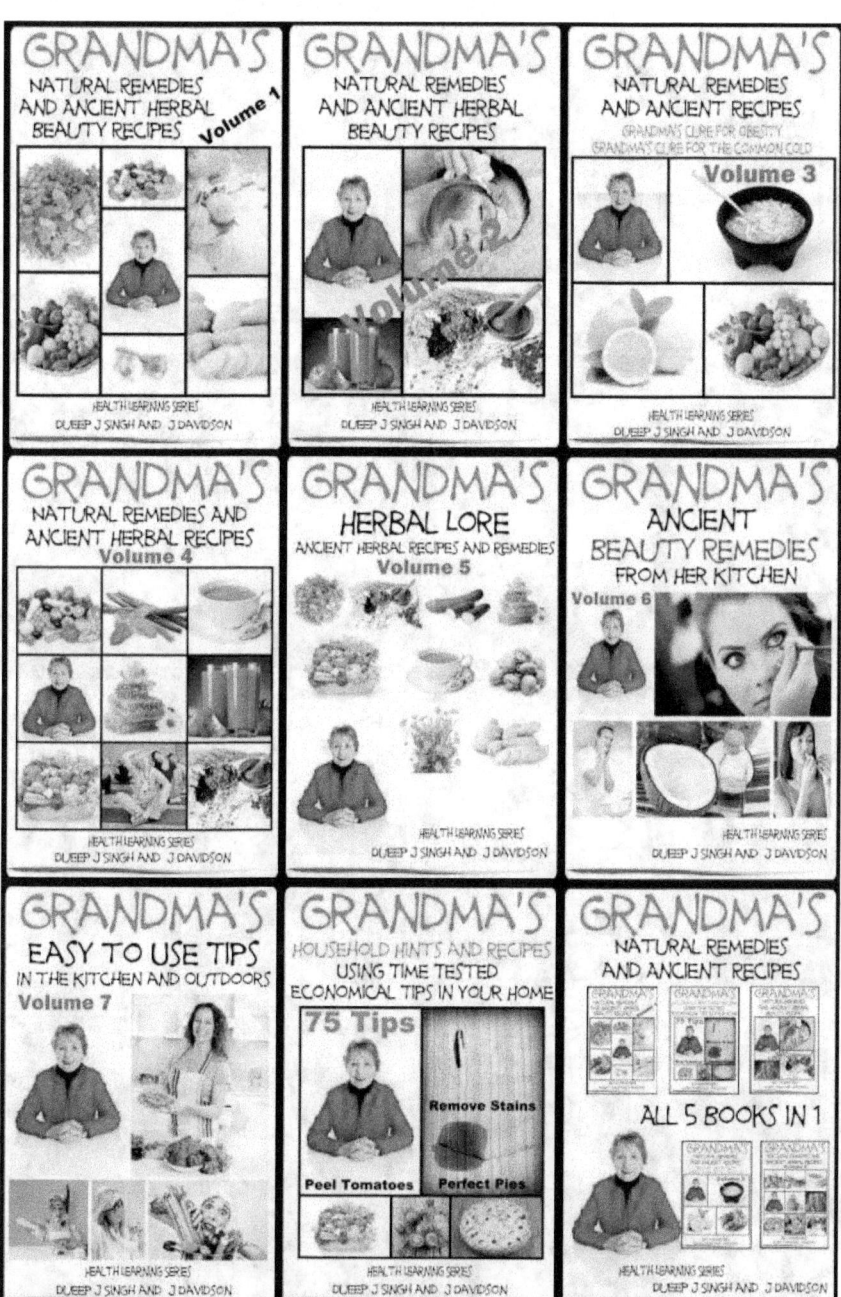

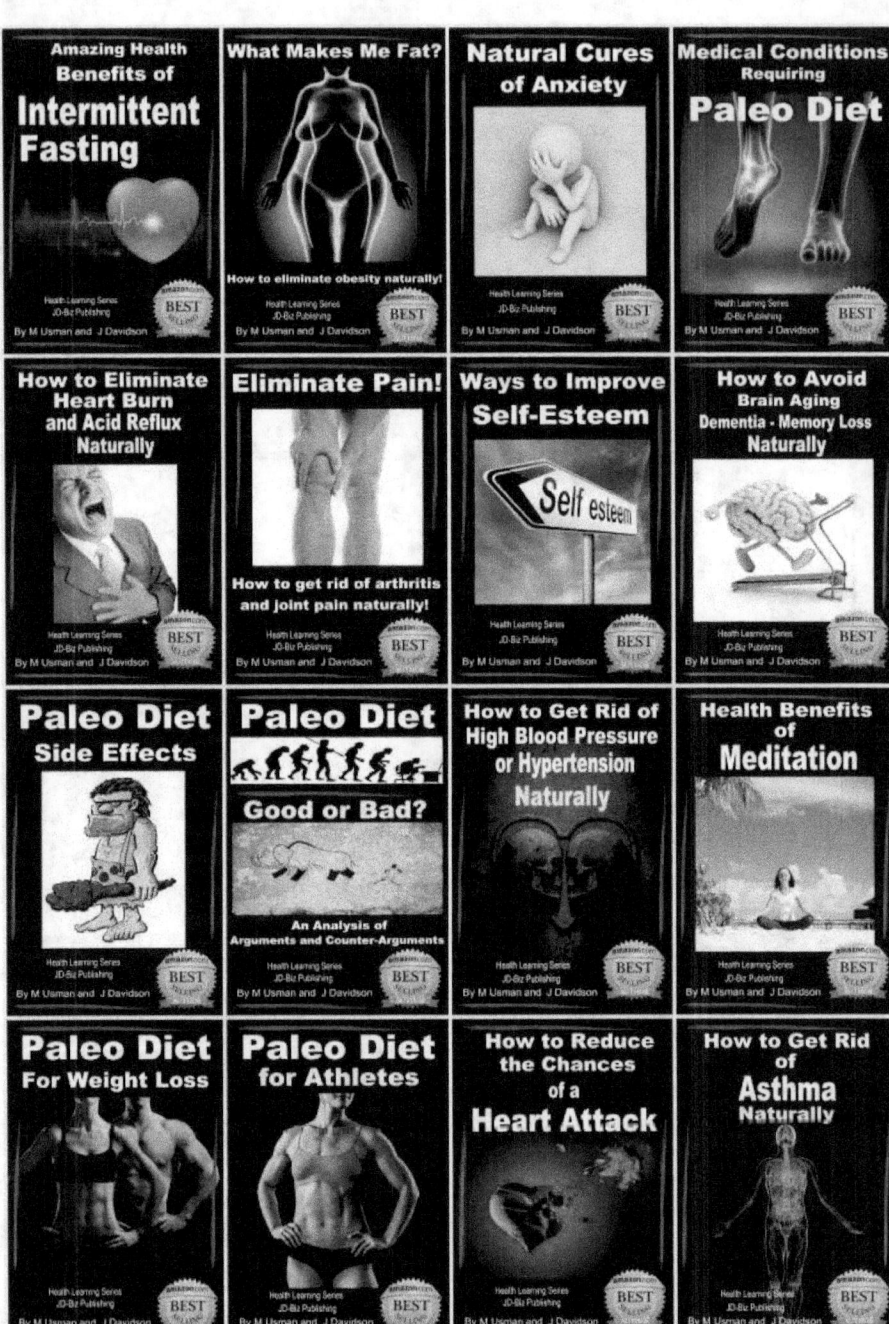

Amazing Animal Book Series

Learn To Draw Series

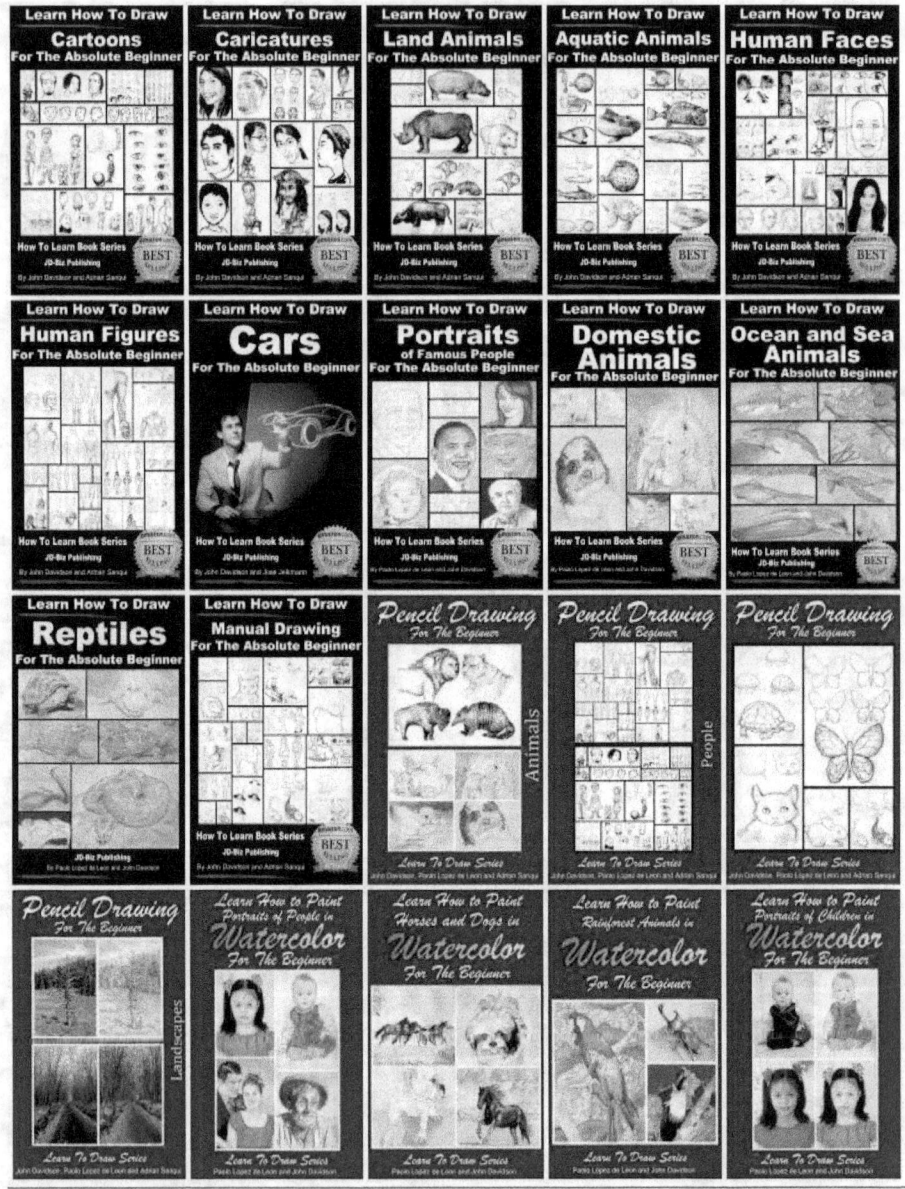

How to Build and Plan Books

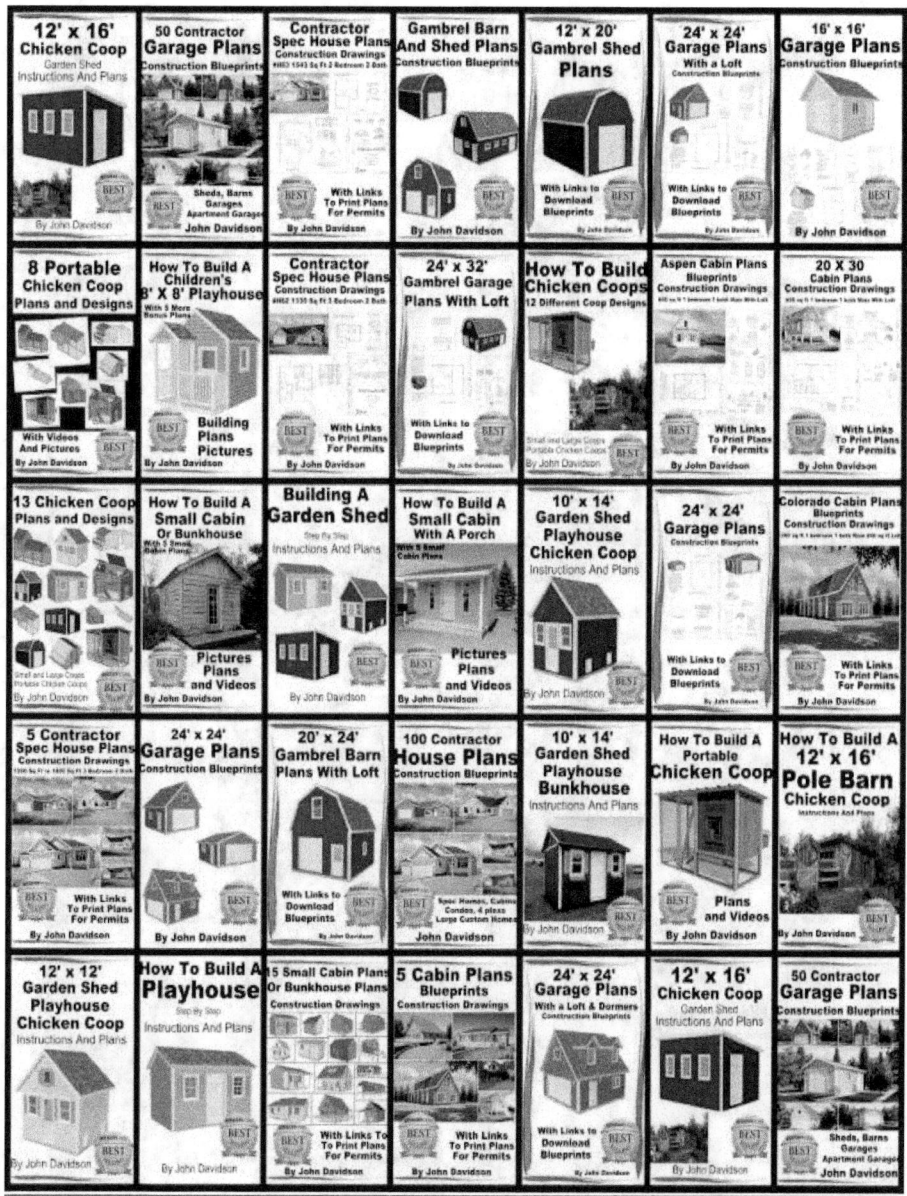

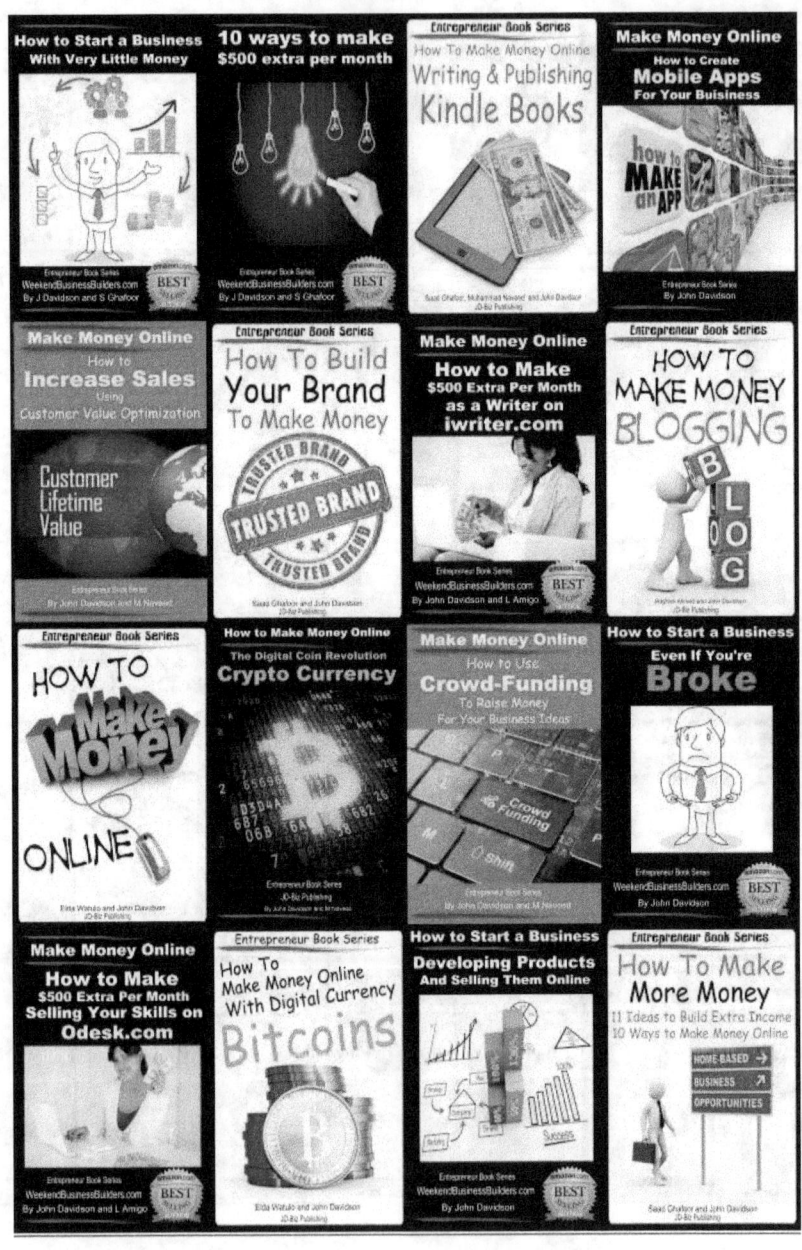

Our books are available at

1. Amazon.com

2. Barnes and Noble

3. Itunes

4. Kobo

5. Smashwords

6. Google Play Books

Download Free Books!

http://MendonCottageBooks.com

Publisher

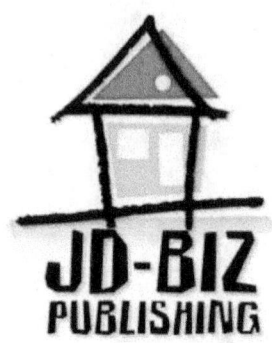

JD-Biz Corp

P O Box 374

Mendon, Utah 84325

http://www.jd-biz.com/

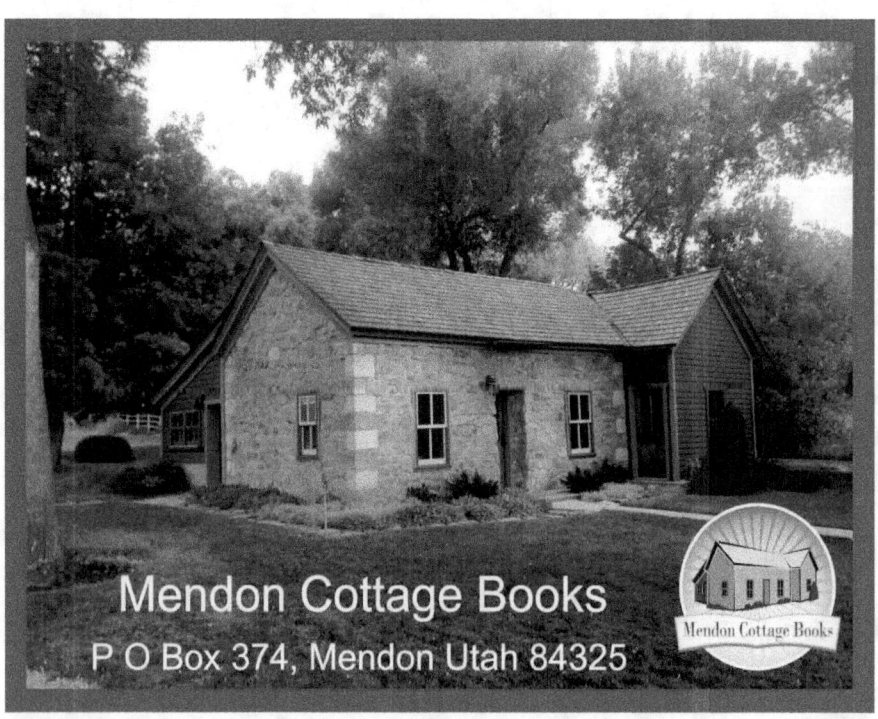

Mendon Cottage Books

P O Box 374, Mendon Utah 84325

www.ingramcontent.com/pod-product-compliance
Lightning Source LLC
Chambersburg PA
CBHW071134280526
45787CB00003B/1279